"Beth Gainer's book, *Calling the Shots in Your Medical Care*, is a must-read for every patient and caregiver. Written with a straightforward and compelling voice, Gainer offers sound advice to get the best medical care. She should know. She is a breast cancer survivor who lived through and overcame many challenges in her medical journey.

Calling the Shots in Your Medical Care focuses on the all-important doctor-patient relationship, showcasing that the quality of that relationship is the cornerstone of good medical care. Through interesting stories, Gainer illustrates how to find a truly great doctor and which behaviors to look for. Through her experiences, we recognize arrogant doctors who don't listen to patients, those who aren't interested in patient-centered care.

Calling the Shots in Your Medical Care is both an emotional and captivating read. It is packed with effective strategies for patients to get the best care while maintaining their sanity."

— **Martine Ehrenclou, MA,** author of *The Take-Charge Patient* and *Critical Conditions*.

"Applause to Beth Gainer for her gutsy approach to getting optimal healthcare. In this straightforward volume, she gives direct advice to patients regarding choosing, monitoring, and partnering your own healthcare team. Also, she speaks frankly and wisely about such crucial issues as how to keep yourself safe in hospital, how to deal with bumbling administration, and how to speak to the arrogant. Examples from her own challenges provide powerful insight into the truth and courage of her approach. Her concept of "civil disobedience" as a means to patient safety is both correct and compelling. As I read it, I kept thinking, 'If only I had read this before my own health debacle.' Many people will be empowered, and perhaps even saved, by this pithy and punchy book."

— **Robin McGee**, author of *The Cancer Olympics*

"*Calling the Shots in Your Medical Care* is an urgently needed guide for people who are learning to advocate for themselves in a complicated medical world. It is all too easy to feel disempowered, frightened, and even pushed into uncomfortable decisions about caretakers as well as treatments. Ms. Gainer gives us a straightforward primer that teaches patients how to endorse their own values while securing the best possible medical care. Do yourself a favor and read this book."

— **Hester Hill Schnipper,** LICSW, BCD, OSW-C, Program Manager Oncology Social Work Beth Israel Deaconess Medical Center, Boston, MA, and the author of *After Breast Cancer: A Common-Sense Guide to Life After Treatment*

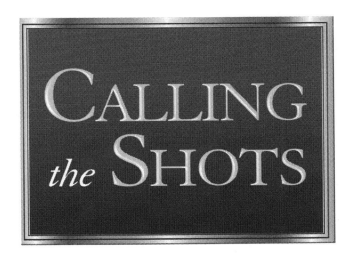

CALLING *the* SHOTS

in Your
Medical Care

Beth L. Gainer, MA

Medical disclaimer: This book does not offer professional medical advice and cannot substitute for proper medical care.

Published by

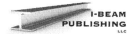

Chicago, IL.

Gainer, Beth L.
Calling the Shots in Your Medical Care: Beth L. Gainer. – 1st edition
      1. Self Advocacy
      2. Medical Care
      3. Patient
      4. Illness
      5. Caregiver
      6. Gateway Doctor

Book cover and interior design by
Deborah Perdue of Illumination Graphics

Library of Congress Control Number: 2016936164

ISBN -10: 0-9968-2530-4
ISBN-13: 978-0-9968-253-0-6
FIRST EDITION

Printed in the United States of America

Dedication

*This book is dedicated to my
readers who, at some time or
another, must call the shots
in their own medical care.*

Beth L. Gainer

Acknowledgments

I WANT TO THANK THE GIFTED AND BRILLIANT people who helped me with this book: Robin Scholz, you have helped me beyond measure with your precise editing that has enhanced my book; Cynthia Morris, of Original Impulse Inc., for coaching me through the difficult emotional process of writing *Calling the Shots in Your Medical Care*; and Deborah Perdue of Illumination Graphics, OR, for exquisite book design work.

A special thanks to my first writing coach Roger Bresnahan, professor at Michigan State University. You encouraged a nervous college freshman to become a confident writer.

Thank you to my family and friends who have spent time listening to my story and who gave their support while I was going through medical crises and while I was writing this book. In particular, thanks to my dear friend Judith Rhodes; you have continued to encourage and support my dream to make this book a reality.

I want to thank Dr. Sandy Goldberg, fellow breast cancer survivor and founder of A Silver Lining Foundation (www.asilverliningfoundation.org), a wonderful organization that advocates for underserved individuals in the breast health arena. You have inspired me each day you do good in the world, which is every day. I have appreciated your support and friendship over the years.

Finally, I want to thank my wonderful daughter, Arielle Gainer, who has always known how important it has been for mommy to share her story and help others.

Table of Contents

Foreword

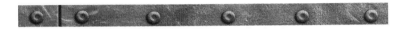

I MET BETH GAINER THROUGH A MUTUAL acquaintance. As breast cancer survivors we bonded immediately as members of a club no one wants to join. Our connection was instantaneous – as both of us understood our good fortune at having access to health care and, most importantly, we had the right to advocate for our own health.

Self-advocacy is not at the forefront of our thinking until forced into a situation where the information we receive does not jive with that little voice in our head saying "Wait a minute here; something doesn't seem quite right." That can stem from feeling as though our questions and opinions don't matter (how can we question traditional medicine as laypeople) and we are left wanting. Beth refused to step to the side: when her questions were not answered, when she felt as though she was not being listened to she sprang into action, advocating for herself and ultimately the thousands of women and men who will read her book. Written by a patient for a patient, this book has the potential to significantly impact the reader's life. The patient bill of rights – so simple yet so far reaching.....that alone will make each and every one sit up and take notice and say "I matter. I can ask questions. The words of someone who does not know me and recognize that I take care of myself should and must be taken into account." Yet, Beth's book is not inflammatory; her concern is educating individuals to speak for themselves.

Self-advocacy and self-empowerment go hand in hand. Having a skill set to deal with an increasingly impersonal medical system is at the heart of this book. I cannot recommend it more highly.

Dr. Sandy Goldberg, Founder of A Silver Lining Foundation, Chicago, IL, and former NBC5's on air Nutrition Contributor

I saved my own life twice.

The first time was when I found my own breast cancer through a routine monthly breast self-exam and brought it to my doctor's attention.

The second time I insisted on a preventive double mastectomy with reconstruction to reduce my chances of recurrence. Biopsy results revealed that one of my "healthy" breasts was filled with precancerous cells.

It turns out, in a formidable medical system, I proved a formidable self-advocate – by calling the shots in my own medical care. Had I not advocated for myself, you would not be reading this book.

You, too, can call the shots in your medical care.

Here's how.

Introduction

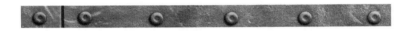

THIS SHORT BOOK IS DESIGNED TO ENCOURAGE
and inspire you to take the reins of your own medical care.
Whether you have advocated for your or a loved one's
health, or you want to know how to do so, this book is for
you. If you have no health problems, you are lucky, but
you also need this book. What better time to line up
excellent physicians than when you are healthy?

I became a self-advocate when I was diagnosed with breast
cancer in January 2001. The road toward health has been
fraught with difficulties, setbacks, losses, and suffering, but I
am grateful to be alive and loved, and to have a platform
through which I can help others. Every person who is
diagnosed with any medical condition is unlucky. In
particular, the word "cancer" fills people's hearts with dread.

In some respects, I was especially unlucky when I was
diagnosed with breast cancer at a young age. I suffered

through three lumpectomies, chemotherapy and radiation, constant medical testing, a few terrifying false alarms, and eventually a preventive double mastectomy with reconstruction. I also became infertile as a result of the treatments. The ironic part of it all is that prior to my diagnosis I was in excellent shape and fit – or so I thought. But despite my diagnosis, I was also lucky: I hired excellent doctors, and I had the best advocate in the world – myself.

Through self-advocacy, I caught my own breast cancer, prevented a recurrence, and ensured I received top-quality HMO medical care. Before my breast cancer diagnosis, I knew nothing about interacting with doctors and self-advocacy. Sure, I had routine exams, but like many people, I was intimidated by doctors and believed everything they told me. I was not immersed in the medical world. My breast cancer experience would change all that.

Throughout my journey of self-advocacy, I have taken actions that were unthinkable to my pre-cancer self: hiring and firing doctors, asserting my needs to medical personnel, scolding difficult medical staff – and in one instance – allowing everyone on a train car to know my sordid, private medical details! Regardless of your condition, situation, prognosis, or ultimate outcome, too much is at stake to allow organizations and medical personnel to intimidate you and fully determine your fate.

You are the one who calls the shots in your own medical care.

During my public speaking engagements, people often ask my advice on how to find the right physician, what to do if they are unhappy with their doctors, or how to handle being dismissed by medical personnel. Patients need to know how to advocate for themselves. *This book does not offer professional medical advice and cannot substitute for proper medical care.* Instead, the book offers tips and techniques to help you take an active role in your medical care and make decisions that are best for *you*. While I use examples of my own self-advocacy experiences, no two experiences are alike, as no two patients are alike. This book focuses on helping you advocate for yourself.

Although you cannot always control your medical situation, remember this: *you* are the driver of your medical care, not a passenger. When it comes to self-advocacy, *you* call the shots.

Note to Caregivers: If you are caring for a person who somehow is too afraid or unable to speak up for him/herself, please act on his/her behalf. Is it difficult? Yes. But not speaking up for the patient can have detrimental consequences. Be courageous. You, too, can be the ordinary person who does the extraordinary. Feel free to take the above advice and speak up to receptionists or any other medical personnel who you feel have not respected the patient. You are more powerful than you know.

It is true that your continued or future health is not always in your control. However, taking charge of your medical care can help you do the seemingly unthinkable – make a challenging medical system work for *you*. You can do this, even in the landscape of managed care and bureaucracies.

Doctors, their staff, and medical offices can be so intimidating that patients forget how much power they have. That's right: Even in the direst situations, you have enormous power to make the medical system work in your favor, persevere through setbacks and hassles, and overcome your fears and act in spite of them.

Unfortunately, too many patients view doctors as being at the top of the hierarchy in the doctor-patient relationship. This is a mistake. No doubt, physicians are knowledgeable resources who play a huge role in caring for patients. However, patients should be collaborators in their health care. In fact, a diagram illustrating the patient-doctor relationship should look something like this:

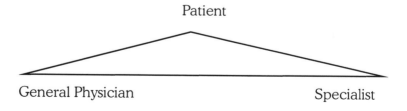

Patient

General Physician   Specialist

Note that patients are at the apex of the triangle: they really are the ones with the power and the final say on medical decisions or which doctors to hire and fire. If doctors are in charge, that's only because patients allow them to be. Many doctors would disagree with me and say that the doctor knows what's best for patients. But that is completely untrue. Only patients really know what's best for patients. And you are the one to determine whether a physician is a good fit for you.

Some physicians like passive patients. You want to choose the doctors who encourage their patients to have a say in their own medical care. You want to listen to their advice, as well as feel free to draw your own medically sound conclusions based on doctors' knowledge. By collaborating with the doctor, you can both create a self-care plan.

It seems as if the burden is on you, the patient. It is.

Let's face it: self-advocacy is difficult and frustrating, requiring you to tap deep within your courage bank to motivate yourself to take action and overcome setbacks. You must be willing to make tough decisions and question medical staff, which is not always popular with those in the medical field.

If you are reading this, you are strong enough to determine what's best for you and to advocate for yourself. You have enormous power, and this book will help you unleash it.

Gutsy Instincts: My Story

The First Time I Saved My Own Life

MY ROUTINE MAMMOGRAM IS NEGATIVE, BUT the report troubles me: It says my breasts are highly dense – common for young people – and therefore, could be somewhat inconclusive. A recent breast exam at my gynecologist's office reveals no abnormalities. I allow myself to be lulled into joyful complacency. And I let my guard down.

A few months later, I am performing my routine breast self exam. I can't feel anything abnormal, but I see something unusual in the mirror: a small dimple at the very top of my right breast.

Could it be cancer? I deny it for two weeks, telling myself that test results and doctors' breast exams are always accurate. But my intuition keeps gnawing at me, so I insist my gynecologist re-examine that breast. He dismisses the dimple as nothing, but he refers me to my hospital's breast center for a diagnostic mammogram, just to be on the safe side.

Once again I rejoice, this time at my gynecologist's confidence I don't have breast cancer, but during my diagnostic mammogram I panic when the mammography technician takes many, many X-rays of my right breast. The radiologist tells me that the mammogram has found a barely visible mass in my right breast, but the abnormality could be benign. Weeks later, while I'm waiting for my biopsy results, several doctors reassure me that I am too young for breast cancer, and the odds are in my favor.

But, as it turns out, I have breast cancer. My world is shattered. I choose a lumpectomy and follow my oncologist's advice to get chemotherapy and radiation simultaneously. I'm sick as hell.

But I'm alive.

Had I chosen complacency instead of acting *in spite of* my fears, the malignancy would've gone undetected – and you would not be reading this book.

The Second Time I Saved My Life

I have just hit my five-year survival mark, the well-known cancer milestone. Because I almost slipped through the medical cracks prior to diagnosis, I get annual MRIs in addition to mammograms. When my oncologist calls me with the test results, I expect him to tell me – as he always tells me – that the results look good.

But instead, he sounds awkward, sorry, and bewildered. He tells me that the MRI has detected something in the breast affected by cancer a half decade before. "It might not be anything; it could be benign, but we first have to see what it is before we figure out what the next step should be," he says cautiously.

My heart sinks, as I think of a friend who – young like me – died from breast cancer only a few months prior to this call. My oncologist tries to reassure me and then orders an ultrasound on that breast; then my surgeon performs a biopsy. The radiologist tells me the ultrasound reveals nothing conclusive. I have a burning question, and it takes all my courage to ask it: Can he see what's going on in my breast? He responds, "Between your surgeries and dense breast tissue, it's impossible to tell what's going on in your breast." Very unsettling.

Luckily, the biopsy reveals that the mass in question is just scar tissue. My doctors are relieved. But I am not. My intuition tells me that if I keep my dense breasts, I'm likely to slip through the cracks again and get another scare or even a recurrence. Against the advice of several doctors, and with the support of key ones, I have a preventive double mastectomy with reconstruction.

But the road toward the double mastectomy is a long one, filled with frustration, unexpected challenges, and lots of hard work dealing with doctors and the medical system. It is what helps me become an even better self-advocate. *I am going to determine my own fate, not just complacently wait for another scare or actual cancer.*

I am proactive.

And with good reason, for a biopsy on my post-mastectomy breast tissue reveals that my left breast, my supposedly always-healthy breast, was filled with precancerous cells. My oncologist tells me that had I not gotten the double mastectomy, I would most likely have gotten cancer again. My decision to get the surgery was a sound one. I realize how very important it is to know my body, follow my gut instincts, and act in spite of my fears. I also realize that while doctors know about the human body, that doesn't mean they know about *my* body. I saved my own life, thanks to my doctors, and mostly thanks to me.

So I discovered that self-advocacy is a crucial part of self-care. And I decided to write this book to help you both cope and avoid the all-too-common pitfalls in navigating your way through the medical system.

Patient-Centered Bill of Rights

Too often, patients are confused by the language of various 'Patient's Bills of Rights' because the language is often convoluted and confusing. It's hard enough to be a patient, so reading through muddling language only adds anxiety.

So here's *my* version of what a Patient's Bill of Rights should look like:

PATIENT'S BILL OF RIGHTS

1. You have the right to be civilly disobedient with any medical personnel who you perceive does not have your best interest at heart.

2. You have the right to hire and fire doctors at will.

3. You have the right to question treatments without a doctor being condescending to you.

4. You have the right to understand you are on equal footing with a doctor because you are both human beings with comparable self-worth.

5. You have the right to collaborate with excellent doctors you trust and who truly have your best interest at heart.

---

6. You have the right to a voice in your own medical care.

7. You have a right to have doctors return your phone calls on a timely basis.

8. You have the right to follow your gut instinct and not allow medical people to manipulate you into ignoring it.

9. Whether you are incapacitated, in the hospital, or extremely sick, you have the right to speak up in any medical settings.

10. You have the right to choose your medical destiny to whatever extent possible.

11. You have the right not to be bullied or badgered by anyone – from receptionist to doctor – at any time.

12. You have the right to be treated with respect and to employ civil disobedience if you are being bullied, badgered, and disrespected in any way. In short, say "no" to thugs.

Part I:
HIRING AND FIRING DOCTORS

Hiring and Firing Doctors

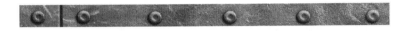

THE FIRST DOCTOR I OFFICIALLY FIRE IS A second-opinion oncologist.

I actually love the oncologist my primary care physician referred me to: he is warm, kind, brilliant, and instantly puts me at ease. I also listen carefully to what nurses and doctors tell me: they'd trust this oncologist with their loved ones' lives. I decide he is the doctor for me.

But I want that damned second opinion. Just because.

Now I am vulnerable again on the examination table, ready to meet Oncologist No. 2. The doctor enters the room with an air of self-importance and arrogance. He talks too rapidly for a frightened patient like me to process. He assaults me with dizzying Internet statistics. In fact, he brings Internet printouts. He flippantly weighs my odds of survival and treatment protocols. He keeps changing his mind. I can't understand what he is saying and feel intimidated, diminished, and powerless. He then tries to bully me into selecting his treatment protocol, a much different one than that of the first oncologist. The second-opinion doctor tells me that if I don't choose his treatment protocol – and quickly – that I will die.

I leave his office crying.

The next day, I tell the second-opinion doctor that I am choosing another physician and undergoing a different treatment protocol. He warns me once again of my impending death. Despite my anguish, I fire him anyway. It turns out that Dr. Second Opinion Guy is wrong about my prognosis, treatment, and everything in between. Hiring the first oncologist is the right choice for me. Even while facing a life-or-death situation, I could still be level-headed enough to tell the difference between a physician who cared about my welfare and one who did not. I learned to speak up rather than give up and succumb to a poor doctor's wishes. I followed my gut instincts to hire the right doctor. And I learned that, in the most stressful medical situations, patients still have the power of choice.

With several tips in tow, you can better distinguish good doctors from the not-so-good ones. Good doctors balance information from their fields of expertise *and* apply this knowledge to help their patients.

Here is a list of reasons to run away from doctors. I have experienced all of these scenarios, some multiple times. If a physician shows one or more of these qualities, consider it a red flag. Great doctors may go on vacation, but never on a power trip.

Time to Run Checklist

Below are the signs that you need to put on your running shoes:

✔ Not listening or allowing you to speak your mind.

✔ Citing one dizzying statistic after another, trying too hard to impress, or making you feel inferior/stupid.

✔ Having a cheat sheet from the Internet and reading from it during an appointment.

✔ Bringing up the removal of organs that are not up for discussion.

✔ Maligning his/her colleagues and taking offense if you want another doctor's opinion.

✔ Blaming you for not taking his/her advice.

✔ Trying to decide your medical destiny rather than act as your advisor when you are the one in charge of your own medical destiny.

✔ Playing God by predicting what will happen to you, when the truth is nobody knows the outcomes for sure, including a physician.

✔ Pressuring you to make decisions too quickly for your comfort level.

The Gateway Doctor

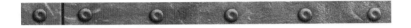

I REALLY LIKE MY GENERAL DOCTOR. WHENEVER I become ill or have a routine exam, she is knowledgeable and treats me with respect. But during my breast cancer diagnosis and prognosis, she turns into a superstar. She often calls me to help coach me through my ordeal. She listens to me and validates my concerns. She encourages questions and provides prompt, thorough answers. She returns my phone calls immediately. And while I am obsessed with breast cancer and panicking, she is level-headedly working behind the scenes, putting an excellent team in place for me. She lands me a great surgeon and a fantastic medical oncologist.

These exceptional professionals all work tirelessly to save my life, but they don't treat me as if I am a patient. They treat me like family. And they are HMO doctors, dispelling the myth that all HMOs are poor. My specialists are unbelievably outstanding and kind – like off-the-charts brilliant and sweet people. Had it not been for my general physician, or "gateway doctor," I know I never would have crossed paths with them.

Having a great general physician in place was paramount in my medical care. Even though I felt my life was spinning out of control with my breast cancer diagnosis, I felt some control that I had hired the right general doctor to begin with. One can never overestimate the importance of such a physician.

Besides you, the most important person managing your health care is the "gateway doctor," also known as the primary care physician (PCP), internist, general family doctor, and so on. An excellent gateway physician makes decisions on whatever is in *your* best interest, not the interest of health-management corporations.

A huge perk of a great gateway physician is that he or she tends to keep company with other excellent doctors, and that opens the gateway to outstanding specialists and first-rate medical care. Whether or not you are healthy, whether or not your family has had the same physician they have felt comfortable with for decades, whether or not your doctor is well-versed in all of the new medical technologies, whether or not your doctor has had an established practice with a good reputation, it all boils down to this:

Do you trust your family doctor with your life?

If the answer is anything but a resounding, enthusiastic "YES!," find another doctor immediately. Your life is too precious to take a chance with mediocrity and, even worse, total incompetence. I measure competent doctors by their medical *and* emotional know-how. They must be medically competent (It sounds like I'm stating the obvious, but it needs to be stated), *and* they must have your best interest at heart. The latter point means more than just bedside manner: I have had doctors be pleasant to me, but mere pleasantries are not enough reason to choose a physician.

You must LOVE your doctor.

The ideal gateway doctor cares about you as a patient and will work as hard as possible to advocate for you. I was lucky to have an outstanding gateway doctor in place before I got diagnosed with breast cancer. She was my physician for years prior to my diagnosis because we had great patient-doctor chemistry.

You've heard me wax poetic about my gateway doctor. Now it's time to find yours or to see if he or she measures up to your high standards. Here are some litmus tests that can help you find the doctor who is right for you. These tests also apply to specialists, but you often need a great general physician in place before you can even consider a specialist.

To find the right physician, the first thing to do is to set up exams, perhaps with several doctors. You need to be patient and have a great deal of resilience to attend several appointments in a relatively short time span. Be creative: go to one doctor for a headache, another for a backache, another for a routine examination, and so on. Trust me, perseverance pays off.

Use the following litmus tests to assess whether a particular doctor is the right one for you.

> **Litmus test one:** During your meeting, give an emotional prompt, like: "I'm afraid of blood tests" or "I'm worried about my cholesterol levels." Observe the doctor's reactions. If the doctor is empathetic and great at putting you at ease, that's an excellent sign. Is he/she emotionally vested in you? Does he or she listen – I mean really listen – to your concerns? Reassuring? If not, find another doctor.

> **Litmus test two:** Sometime in the week following your exam, call the doctor to ask a question. Does the doctor call you back promptly? Does he or she communicate with you clearly and patiently? Does he or she take your concerns seriously? If the answer to any of these is "no," find another doctor.

> **Litmus test three:** Does the doctor play "ring around the patient," continuously throwing

statistics around to impress you with his or her know-how? Does he or she come with print-outs of pages from the Internet to illustrate these statistics? Do you feel confused during and/or after the session? Run – do not walk – away from this doctor.

Litmus test four: Does the doctor use scare tactics, telling you all the terrible things that can happen to you? Is he/she dismissive of your emotional and physical needs? Does he or she sound like a doctor who has watched too many medical-show episodes? If so, this is not the doctor for you.

Litmus test five: Does the doctor rush you through the appointment? Do you feel he or she has no patience with you and/or your questions? If so, then rush out the door and get another doctor.

Litmus test six: Does the doctor answer your questions to your satisfaction and thoroughly – in a way you can understand it? Does he/she mind if you ask questions or take notes? If so, this doctor has issues.

Litmus test seven: Observe the doctor's body language. See if the doctor maintains excellent eye contact, and when you bring up your concern, whether he/she seems in a rush or simply sits down and talks with you. Is the physician distant from you emotionally and physically? If the doctor is comfortable being physically close to you while answering questions, that's a good sign.

Litmus test eight: Cross-examine your doctor by repeating your questions (but not *ad nauseum*) and rewording the questions differently, so you can get consistent answers. If the doctor answers your questions to your satisfaction, this is a good sign.

Based on all these litmus tests, do you LOVE your doctor? If you are feeling badly about him/her, or just so-so, find another physician. Don't settle for mediocrity because if there were a medical crisis, a doctor you love and who cares deeply about your welfare will be the one who fights for you.

The bottom line is never put up with abusive doctors or those who make you feel guilty, marginalized, or insignificant.

You *are* significant.

The main thing is to trust your instincts and be persistent in your goals to find a great doctor. You will know whether a physician is a good fit for you. Also, if you suspect something is wrong, and he or she does not give you a satisfactory answer or solution, then continue advocating for yourself. Don't accept answers like, "You are too young to get cancer" or "You are too young to have heart problems." Demand to be treated with respect and, if necessary, be difficult to those who treat you unfairly. You have an amazing power to garner respect – whether from doctors, nurses, or office personnel. If someone treats you with disrespect, talk back.

You are nobody's doormat, and they need to know it.

A great gateway doctor is a must. If you do not have a doctor you connect with and trust, please find one as soon as possible. My grandmother always told me, "If you have your health, you have everything." As a child, I didn't understand what she meant. I didn't heed her words as a healthy young adult: I came from very genetically healthy stock – people in my family die of old age for goodness sakes, even the ones exposed to asbestos, lead, and various other toxins! But her words resonated with me when I was diagnosed with breast cancer. Luckily, I had an outstanding gateway physician in place at the time. Now I'm going to spin my grandma's words to suit my self-advocacy philosophy: "If you have your health *and* a great gateway doctor, you have everything."

Creating a
Gateway Doctor Menu

I STRONGLY RECOMMEND BECOMING FAMILIAR with most of the doctors in your physicians' group. This way, when your favorite doctor isn't available, you can choose another doctor whom you trust. When Plan A doesn't work, Plan B should. And Plan B involves thinking of the available doctors as items on a menu and helps you choose the best doctor at your specific time of need.

Generally, it's a good idea to think of general doctors in a particular practice as menu items. Just as there are many choices on a restaurant menu – some more preferable to others – there are many doctors from which to choose. Specialists are more tricky because in any one medical group, for example, you might have a select few. But a great gateway physician will more often than not refer you to great specialists.

If you have an HMO, you should know the general doctors who comprise your medical group. If you have a PPO, you need to know about the quality of various networks and key doctors within these networks. If you are uninsured or underinsured, you can research organizations that offer assistance with medical care and, still, you can *demand* competent doctors.

If you are sick or need an exam when your general physician is not available, you should have an arsenal of other choices at your disposal. As mentioned earlier, knowing which doctors you prefer means potentially making appointments with several of these doctors over a course of time. While time-intensive and tedious, this approach can help you best distinguish the doctors you like from the doctors you don't.

Trust me, I practice what I preach. For example, once when I was suffering from bronchitis I called my doctor's office to get an immediate appointment with my primary care physician. To my disappointment, she was not in the office that day. However, the receptionist informed me that several doctors were available, and she seemed taken aback when I asked for the names of all the available doctors, as I was familiar with almost all of them in my group.

Truth be told, I viewed them as if they were items on a menu. The receptionist and I went down the list of available physicians. They were all competent, but my criteria for doctors included their personalities and how they had treated me during prior exams. One available doctor was abusive to me, so I had already fired him. I told the receptionist that I didn't want to use him; another doctor was depressing to deal with, so I told the receptionist, "No thanks, go on with the available doctors." Eventually, we found the right one; I remembered that he helped me at a crucial time when I was hospitalized, and he was kind to me. At the hospital, not only did he order the medication I needed right away, but he made a point to come to my room to meet me and shake my hand. I set up my appointment with him and was pleased. He prescribed the right medication and had a nice demeanor, just as I had expected.

Caveat: Sometimes doctors seem right at a certain time, but then they change and/or you change and this relationship is no longer a fit.

Finding and Hiring
a Great Specialist

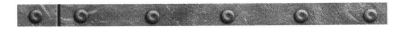

TO FIND A GREAT SPECIALIST, USE THE SAME LITMUS tests you used to find your general physician. When you have an outstanding specialist in place, you can eventually use him or her as your gateway to other specialists. Notice that I said an "outstanding" doctor because nothing less is acceptable.

My oncologist meets – actually exceeds – all the aforementioned criteria. When I need a referral to a specialist, therefore, I now can call my medical oncologist for a recommendation and get my primary care physician to write the referral for the recommended specialist. My oncologist is an extraordinary, brilliant doctor, yet down to Earth. He also returns ALL my calls in a matter of a few hours, sometimes in minutes, even when he's away from the office.

For those of you who think this type of doctor is a rarity, you are right. However, with persistence, checking out a variety of specialists, and by asking questions, you can find such a doctor. While my oncologist's word is generally good as gold, I know that, at the end of the day, I'm the one who has to make the decision about whether a specialist is good. But it sure helps to have an excellent specialist gateway doctor on your side.

Remember this: Great doctors keep company with other great doctors.

It is true. My excellent gateway physician referred me to an outstanding general surgeon and medical oncologist. My outstanding medical oncologist connected me to a wonderful radiation oncologist, mastectomy surgeon, reconstructive surgeon, physical therapist, psychotherapist, gynecologist, and my daughter's pediatrician. And when I asked my oncologist whom he would recommend to do my colonoscopy, he referred me to the doctor who performed his!

Throughout my years as a patient, I continued to hire the doctors who listened and took me seriously. The ones who demeaned me by talking down to me or mistreating me – well, they were so fired. I cannot emphasize the importance of doctors who listen to their patients. Doctors who dismiss their patients' concerns are worth firing.

Remember this: Despite all the business deals to be had, there's no business more important than the hiring and firing of doctors. Your health – and possibly your life – depends on it.

Hiring and Firing Doctors

Hiring Doctors

YOU LOVE A DOCTOR AND DECIDE TO USE HIM OR her. It's as simple as that. Using your litmus tests of finding a gateway doctor or a specialist, you know this doctor is for you. In more specialized circumstances – like after you have met with a bunch of loser doctors – you can reveal during your interview that you are looking for that special doctor. For example, during the final planning of my double mastectomy, I had the reconstruction surgeons lined up, but I needed a mastectomy surgeon.

The first thing I said to her was this: "I've got all my doctors in place – except one. I need someone to do the mastectomy. I'm hoping you are the missing link." She laughed and said she hoped she was, too, and it turned out she was also a breast cancer survivor who happened to have a mastectomy – she really understood where I was coming from. In addition, she was sweet, kind, and empathetic. I hired her on the spot and *told* her she was hired.

Firing Doctors

I could tell you that I yelled at a doctor and pointed at him/her, saying "You're fired!" as I stormed out of the office, but that would be false. Truth is, it's always been really difficult and painful for me to keep from crumbling under the weight of a physician's authority. As a patient, it is easy to be bullied into compliance.

Firing doctors is no easy task. Each time I fired a physician I experienced heartache and even made a discovery that my mascara wasn't waterproof. You will notice that, except for a couple of examples, "firing" meant simply walking away.

Here are just some ways I fired doctors:

1. The surgeon who was so great to me during diagnosis and prognosis, but years later claimed it was unethical to do a preventive mastectomy: I flat-out told him he was wrong and that my gut instinct was right. He sneered at me, and I told him I was using another doctor.

2. The gynecologist who lied to me when I was in my first trimester of pregnancy. Because he wanted to

see me happy, he told me there was a 99.5% chance I'd carry this baby to term. After my post-miscarriage D&C and follow-up, I never went back to this physician.

3. The gynecologist who scolded me for *my* medical decision not to follow his advice. I left the office crying, but I never came back.

4. Oh, and let's not forget that second-opinion oncologist who told me that if I didn't submit to his treatment, I'd be dead in a year – causing me to leave yet another doctor's office crying. I eventually told him I would not take his advice and I was seeing another doctor.

5. One surgeon mocked me for having the audacity to pursue a surgery he didn't agree with.

6. I also fired the doctor who refused to return my calls for a month. And the doctor who scolded me for not wanting to have my ovaries and uterus removed. And the doctor who insisted I not have my breasts removed.

I have to see an enormous number of doctors to determine what procedure is best for me, and which surgeons are lucky enough to be on my team. Some are your garden-variety quacks, freaks, and egomaniacs, all of whom I fired.

While my decisions to hire and fire physicians sound so simple, they are not. This is a very time-consuming, emotional process. It is difficult to be treated poorly by doctors who are arrogant, and it takes a lot of determination not to give up. I almost gave up on my goal for a double mastectomy with reconstruction more times than I can remember. But something within me wouldn't allow it. I kept pushing toward my goal and never gave up.

These examples illustrate a very simple truth: we all have the capacity to advocate for ourselves and that firing doctors need not be dramatic. In fact, sometimes the most courageous acts involve quietly walking away.

In addition, be wary of any doctor who tells you that you are too young for certain conditions. Young people get sick, and a visit to any children's hospital should humble the most dismissive of doctors.

Monitoring Those
Who Monitor You

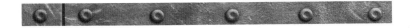

MY FRIEND REALIZES AT THE BEGINNING OF A
chemotherapy treatment that the bag of chemicals
beginning to drip into her body has another patient's name
on it. Horrified, my friend alerts the nursing staff and insists
that this treatment be stopped immediately. Had she not
advocated for herself, she would not only have had the
wrong chemical cocktail as part of her chemotherapy
treatment; she might have died prematurely.

I am luckier. My chemotherapy nurse doesn't make any
mistakes with me. But she admits that because she is
dyslexic, she has to double- and triple-check the
doctors' orders for all patients. We joke about this at
times, but deep down inside, I know to kindly – but
assertively – ensure I am getting the right chemo
treatment. So I ask my chemotherapy nurse, "So what's
the name of this chemical?" and "And which chemical

follows?" Knowing which chemical is going into me and when each is being administered is super-empowering. And even though my chemotherapy nurse remembers the injections I am supposed to receive, I feel obligated to remind her or to talk about it during the course of my sitting in the chemo chair. I am polite enough that I don't offend her. However, I realize that even if she were ultrasensitive and I offended her, I still have to act in my best interest.

Even while enduring chemotherapy I was aware of my medical surroundings. I was still able to exert some control over my situation by asking questions and verifying information about my treatment plan. Even if you have outstanding medical personnel, you need to watch them cross their 't's' and dot their 'i's'. In other words, don't be complacent: Carefully watch how your medical care is unfolding. I'm not suggesting looking over everyone's shoulder and venturing into paranoia. What I *am* suggesting, though, is to be vigilant by taking an active role in your treatments. This is accomplished by asking questions, politely telling staff when you think there's an error, and just being aware of information and actions regarding your treatment.

In addition, when test results are sent to physicians, make sure the results are sent to all the doctors you trust. This encourages a team approach – when they all have a copy of your medical records, your doctors can best communicate with each other.

Assessing the Physician's Environment

MY DAUGHTER AND I ARE WAITING A LONG TIME IN the humid, unventilated waiting room. The air is stale. The pediatrician is overbooked, thus the wait. My daughter clutches me tightly amid the mayhem: Patients and staff are yelling at each other. Staff members look disheveled and disorganized. Patients are complaining about doctors not showing up for their appointments. And the billing explanations seem arbitrary.

Not good signs.

In addition, there are no kid-friendly items, no inviting toys or books, no cheerful décor, and no play areas. In fact, the waiting room looks nothing like a pediatrician's office. Overall, the environment is so dismal that I think the roaches want to commit suicide. Finally, my daughter and I are in the examination room. The smug, arrogant pediatrician overcharges me for a 10-minute "exam." He doesn't even use his stethoscope.

A few weeks later finds my daughter and me at my oncologist's recommended pediatrician. Her waiting room is quiet, kid-friendly, and beautiful. The staff is respectful of the patients and each other. There is real compassion to patients' needs, and staff is smiling and friendly. They speak in soft, calm tones and joke with each other. Everyone seems happy. When the pediatrician walks in with a smile and a gentle voice, I *know* she is the one I'm going to hire. This doctor spends one hour with us. She examines my child from head to toe, backwards and forwards.

And she uses a stethoscope.

The pediatrician anticipates and answers my questions before I have a chance to ask them. At the end of the appointment, she asks me if I have any questions and sits down next to us as if we were friends. I am grateful to my oncologist, as he served as a great gateway doctor who paved the way to an outstanding pediatrician. This experience has reinforced the saying "Birds of a feather flock together." Great doctors don't associate with bird brains; great doctors generally know and form a community with other great doctors. With this new pediatrician, I'm glad I got an eagle instead of another vulture.

I found myself in a difficult situation in a hectic medical environment. A poor office environment can be the tell-tale sign of a poor doctor. You can tell a lot about a doctor by his or her staff and the office environment. This is achieved by reading between the signs. One of the ways you can discern whether a doctor is the right fit for you is by listening – that means listening with *all* your senses. Patients often believe that effective listening begins and ends simply with taking notes and voice recording the doctor's visit. While taking notes and recording doctors' explanations can be helpful, they are poor substitutes for effective listening.

At every doctor's appointment you need to read between the signs, which involves using *all* your senses – hearing, smelling, touching, seeing and, yes perhaps even tasting. If the water from the water cooler tastes unpleasant, for example, this could indicate a cleanliness problem. One friend said she fired a pediatrician because a used hypodermic syringe was lying on a countertop in the exam room. The office staff's excuse: they were too busy to clean after the previous appointment.

Whether in the waiting room, examination room, or the doctor's office, you need to be aware of many environmental cues. For example, is the doctor unprofessional and disheveled? Is the waiting room a chaotic environment with disheveled staff? Is there a rank odor? Is the place unkempt? Do staff and patients sound disgruntled? Are patients complaining that the doctor has missed appointments or was responsible for certain mishaps? Are staff disorganized and seem confused? Is it unusually noisy? Do objects in the waiting room feel grimy? Do staff members seem unhappy?

This is what I mean by listening with *all* your senses. Trust your intuition and pay attention to the doctor's environment because this can tell you a lot about the physician and/or the quality of care you most likely will receive.

In addition, the doctor's office environment is not just a physical space but an emotional one created by the physicians and the rest of the office staff. Don't you just hate the stench of a bad attitude? Or a haughty look? Or the taste of humiliation? I realize this may seem like a stretch, but an office's ambience often reflects the quality of care a patient can expect to receive. For example, a friend's doctor didn't like him taking notes and deftly took the notebook from his hand. The physician said he was joking, but my friend didn't perceive this. The physician turned out to be a dud.

Generally speaking, one cannot always judge a book by its cover, but when it comes to medicine, one often can. Next time you go to a doctor's office – any doctor's office – check out the physical and emotional surroundings and staff. Note if the quality of medical care correlates to those surroundings and people. I'll bet it does. Of course, a nice office cannot guarantee top-notch medical care.

Later in the book, I will address how to cope with less-than-stellar administrators, who – like it or not – are key members of a doctor's environment who can affect your medical and emotional well-being, but overall, as a patient, you need to trust your instincts based on listening to what doctors are saying and indicating. You should listen not only to what doctors are saying but *how* they are saying it.

Besides listening with all your senses in a doctor's office, listen to the repetition of doctors' names. What's in a name? Doctors' names come up repeatedly for a reason. My reconstructive surgeons were touted as the best by more physicians than I could count. And the various doctors who recommended them gave me the references. Nurses would brag about them. Medical staff spoke so highly of my radiation and medical oncologists, I felt confident in them.

In addition, pay attention to how your doctors feel about and treat each other, as well as view and treat subordinates. It was clear to me that my medical oncologist and radiation oncologist thought highly of each other and had great camaraderie. The general surgeon and oncologist worked closely together as a team to help me. There was no backstabbing or doubt on the part of one physician toward another. On the other hand, when my medical oncologist disagreed with a wayward gynecologist's plan of action, it was a sure sign that trouble was afoot, and I decided to fire the gynecologist.

If a physician has many facts, but presents them in "doctor speak" so that you cannot understand what he or she is saying, then you want to ask him or her to clarify what he/she means. If the physician cannot or will not, rethink your choice of physicians.

Don't ignore your gut instincts. This can be the difference between empowerment and passivity, between life and death.

Hiring and Firing Doctors Checklist

To choose the best doctor for you, remember to do the following:

✔ Hire a gateway doctor by going to a number of doctor appointments, assessing the red flags, and referring to the aforementioned litmus tests.

✔ Get to know as many general doctors as possible in a particular practice. This will help you make a second, third, or even fourth choice should the gateway doctor you hired not be available.

✔ Know how to hire and how to fire doctors tactfully.

While it's a good idea to trust those entrusted to monitor you, you still need to monitor these particular people to ensure, to the best of your ability, that you are getting the best treatment.

Assess the physical and emotional environment of a doctor's waiting room and office; this includes the morale of the staff.

Part I – Closing Thoughts

It is challenging in this day and age – in fact it was always a challenge – to find the right doctors who have your best interest at heart. Finding the right physician for you and your needs is fraught with obstacles. However, you do have more power than you may realize. Even in the direst of circumstances, you can choose your doctor and the treatment plan that you believe works best for you. Of course, another way to self-empowerment is to achieve physician support, or doctor buy-in.

Part II:
ACHIEVING DOCTOR BUY-IN

Achieving Doctor Buy-in

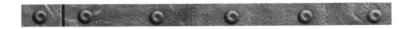

MY ONCOLOGIST SITS DOWN, RESIGNED. I HAVE just informed him I want a preventive double mastectomy with reconstruction. A recent MRI shows a possible recurrence in the same breast that had cancer a few years before. Luckily, a biopsy reveals the mass that the MRI spotted is actually scar tissue. Since cancer, my follow-up mammograms have produced a series of scares. This last one involving the MRI, however, created a sea change: I was now more determined than ever to have my breasts removed.

Now I am facing my oncologist, telling him that enough is enough.

"You are right, you know," he says. "You are likely to slip through the cracks again as long as you have these breasts. Either you will have a recurrence of cancer, or you will keep getting false scares throughout your life."

He tells me he will do whatever he can to support me. We shake hands on the deal, partners in advocacy. Within a few days, he and I separately communicate this plan to my primary care physician. She agrees a preventive double mastectomy with reconstruction is in my best interest. A surgeon agrees my decision is medically sound.

My decision.

And I've achieved doctor buy-in.

Through the process of achieving doctor buy-in, I learned to take a stand for myself. I spoke up and effected change in the course of my care, rather than be silenced by fear of the medical system. I knew how to take care of myself and felt a sense of control in a situation where control was difficult to find.

Great doctors will more than likely give you great medical advice. They look out for your best interest. But a wonderful physician will also be open to the patient's input. He or she will respect your medical decisions – if they are sound. In fact, you should feel comfortable with making sound medical decisions on your behalf. And sometimes this means having doctors write letters on your behalf.

The Letter-Writing Campaign

The right doctor for you is open-minded, on your side, and advocates for your medical needs – in writing if need be.

He or she is therefore willing to write letters on your behalf. If you already have such a doctor in place, you are one step ahead of the game. If your doctors are not open to your reasonable ideas and requests – and I mean *reasonable* – consider finding doctors who are. This is not easy, but it may be necessary.

Once a doctor buys into your reasonable medical vision, then his/her letter becomes crucial in order for you to get the medical care you need and deserve. It seems everyone needs a doctor's letter at some point, whether it tells an insurance company that you need to see an out-of-network specialist, informs an employer to make reasonable accommodations for you so you can work in spite of your medical condition, or proves you are in good health and able to work or adopt a child. The list goes on and on. You can have doctors write letters, you can dictate to doctors what you want the letters to say, or you can ghost write them.

I should know. I've done all three.

Yes, I'm savvy, resourceful, and clever. And so are you.

Most of the time the doctor needs to write the letter, and sometimes the doctor needs you to tell them what you need the letter to say. Don't be afraid to ask a doctor to write a letter on your behalf. This option isn't always first and foremost on doctors' minds. You may need to be bold and make the first move. Don't assume that doctors already know that they should write a letter on your behalf.

Basically, if you can put a sentence together, and your doctor is open-minded, you can ask him or her whether you can write the letter and have him/her read and sign it if he/she agrees with it. When I was going through the process to adopt a child from China, I wrote my doctor's letter to my adoption agency, telling the truth that I was healthy enough to adopt a child. He signed it.

This last point sounds super gutsy, but in reality, with a great doctor, it's relatively simple. Doctors have professional e-mail addresses, and you can e-mail the letter to the physician, and he/she can read it over for accuracy and make whatever changes are needed. Then your doctor prints it out on letterhead, signs it, and sends it to you or the party who is supposed to receive it.

This is a win-win scenario, as you get to control most of the letter's contents, and you've just made life easy for the doctor, who is generally super busy and wants less paperwork.

Caveat: You and your doctor have to know when you can write the letter or when he/she must write it. In addition, you and the doctor should be honest and ethical about your condition/circumstances. Ethical, excellent doctors do exist; you just need to find them. Or perhaps you're lucky enough that you already have one or more. Also assess your ability to write an excellent letter – this approach does not work for everyone.

In addition, getting a doctor to write a note saying it's medically necessary to get a procedure when it really is not medically necessary is unethical. Sure, I would like my skin under my chin to be a bit less droopy, but getting a doctor to write a note that it's medically necessary for me to get plastic surgery would be wrong. Besides, I love my physical imperfections.

The key is to have the right doctors and coverage in place, so if a medical need arises, they will advocate for you.

Achieving Doctor Buy-In Checklist

To achieve doctor buy-in, do the following:

✔ Hire excellent doctors who listen to your input and have your best interest at heart.

✔ When necessary, ask doctors to write letters on your behalf. This is a necessary step, in many cases, to getting the care you need and deserve.

Part II – Closing Thoughts

The relationship between a doctor and patient should be a close one of trust and partnership. You have a strong say in your health care and, if necessary, treatment plan. Achieving doctor buy-in is only one aspect of taking care of yourself. Another way you can care for yourself is to continue to self-advocate – even when you are ill.

Part III:
ADVOCACY
WHEN
SICK

Advocacy When Sick

My Mistake as a Cancer Patient

MY BREAST CANCER TREATMENTS ARE MAKING ME ill. And my biggest mistake when undergoing chemotherapy and radiation is that I don't speak up enough. Ironically, the person who further teaches me to speak up – is of all people – my oncologist. He believes in empowering patients.

While I can't take the blame for the effects the treatments have on me physically and spiritually, I am not being assertive. For example, the anti-nausea medication isn't working, but I don't call my oncologist because I don't want to be any trouble or to be perceived as a whiner. I can't sleep at night because cancer treatments cause my whole digestive system to feel as if it were on fire. Yet I refuse to complain.

Truth is, at this point, doctors still intimidate me somewhat. Plus, I buy into the old model that doctors' decisions are golden and that patients have little, if any, say in their medical care. I wrongly believe that a patient's job is to stoically handle harsh treatments without complaint, lest he or she be considered a chronic complainer. At my next appointment, I casually bring up these issues. My oncologist tells me to speak up and ask for medication to combat the side effects of cancer treatment. He says I would heal better if I could suffer less. He adds adamantly, "If you are sick or something is wrong, then I need to know about it."

A doctor tells me I have the right to complain. I'm shocked.

My oncologist doesn't believe in stifling patients. A great doctor believes in empowering patients and in hearing the truth about how they are feeling. Such a physician listens to his or her patients and encourages them. With my doctor's guidance, I learned to be less passive and to push my self-advocacy forward. To be a patient is to be a collaborator in your medical care. You and the doctor need to work together to figure out what is happening – or not happening – in your body. This doesn't mean that the mystery will be solved, but a doctor's job is to figure out what the problem is, and, if possible, how to remedy it or alleviate it.

Bringing issues to your doctors' attention is *your* job.

Patients don't complain to doctors about treatment-related or illness-/injury-related symptoms for a variety of reasons. Some patients are afraid to royally piss off a doctor. Others often feel they will receive an unsatisfactory response or lack of empathy. A good number of patients do not want to bother the doctor by interrupting his or her daily routine, believing that doctors have more important patients to tend to. However, remember this: there is no more important patient than *you*. So make that call and let the doctor know how you are feeling. A physician isn't a mind reader and cannot help you if you do not speak up about how you are feeling.

Gaining a Sense of Control

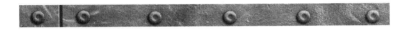

I'M LOSING CONTROL OF MY LIFE.

Doctors and chemotherapy nurses are invading my life. I'm understandably frustrated: These medical professionals are scheduling my time, telling me when and where I'd be getting the next round of treatment, when I'd see a doctor, if I'd see a doctor, when I'm getting blood-work, and so on. I often have to cancel business meetings and put my personal plans on hold, and I am quickly learning that saying "This date won't work for me; can we do the next day?" is futile. The nurse ever-so-nicely says "You *will* be here on this date."

To make matters worse, the treatments are wreaking havoc on my body, as my immune system is no longer working properly, and I have a host of cancer-treatment-related medical problems. My red and white blood cell counts are low, and nothing I do to increase them seems to work. In addition, I have cognitive dysfunction, also known as chemobrain. And while most people I know are supportive, some friends and family reject me – just when I need them the most. In fact, the rejection seems more emotionally trying than the disease itself.

Depression and anxiety set in.

One day my radiation oncologist is on vacation, and, although I love her, I am grateful I won't have to see her. After my radiation treatment, the nurse says, to my shock, "A doctor will see you now." I stammer, "But my doctor is on vacation, and I don't want to see another doctor." Despite my protests, the nurse ushers me into an examining room to wait to see the physician and says nicely, "The doctor will see you soon."

I sob.

The nurse immediately holds me in her arms, wipes away my tears and rocks me like the baby I am. I don't know her name, but I am grateful for her compassion.

What I Learned:

Being a patient with a serious illness meant knowing my life was spinning out of control. However, it's also important to know that seeking and choosing treatment in the first place gives one some sense of control. I learned that a patient has more control than he or she may think. In addition, it's fine to wear your emotions on your sleeve, no matter how raw they are.

Being ill is unnerving and disarming, complicated and difficult. While doctors choose their careers, patients don't choose their careers as patients. Even with a great arsenal of doctors, you most likely will experience a vast array of fears and emotions. It's normal to feel as if your life is spinning out of control.

It is.

Taking Control Checklist

This is when you need to gain some control through the chaos of being a patient. To do this, do the following:

✔ Speak up about feeling poorly. As stated earlier, too many patients – and I have been one of them – try not to "bother" the doctor by complaining about troublesome symptoms, medication side effects, and so on. With your excellent cadre of doctors in place, you should feel comfortable and empowered to talk freely with any physician and any nurse on your team.

✔ Call your doctor with questions. This falls under the not-wanting-to-bother-the-doctor category, as well as a patient's fear of seeming stupid by asking questions. Feel free to ask questions, even if you need to clarify what you had already asked him or her. A great doctor won't mind and will do his or her best to answer your questions to the fullest.

✔ Share your emotional state with medical personnel. It's really important for doctors and other medical staff to see you as a human being who happens to be a patient. Tell doctors and nurses that you feel you no longer have control over your own life. Let your emotions out: cry if you need to, and/or verbalize how you feel emotionally. This should help remind the medical team that you are a real person with real feelings.

This should also remind you how powerful you can be in persuading medical staff to be your champions. Remember that you have the power to do the following:

✔ Fire a doctor who silences you rather than listens to you. A doctor who mistreats you should not be your doctor. Enough said.

✔ Ask the same question in different ways, multiple times. As previously stated, it's often easy to get lost in medical-speak and get confused. That's why it is so crucial to ask questions – even if they are the same questions worded differently – to get a concrete, understandable answer. Sometimes you need to reiterate what a doctor says just to ensure you understand what is being said. Clarifying information is a win-win for everyone on your team.

✔ **Use your pharmacist as advocate.** If a doctor doesn't return your phone calls or he/she gives you unsatisfactory answers regarding medication, all you have to do is phone a friend – your local pharmacist. Not only can a pharmacist explain the side effects of a drug, one is available 24/7.

A pharmacist knows medication information intimately, and every time I have called or seen a pharmacist to double check information on a medication, he/she has known the information by rote memory and logic. That's why he/she specializes in medications. I'm not saying that doctors are incompetent and don't know the answers to your questions on medicines. What I am saying is that if you receive a confusing or unsatisfactory answer from a doctor or just happen to be waiting a long time for a callback, consider a pharmacist.

✔ **Use a toolbox to cope in the waiting and examination room.** Like many, if not all of you, I've spent long times waiting in the examination room for the doctor to arrive. When the wait is short, it's sweet. When the wait is long, well....

We will discuss waiting in the waiting and examination rooms in a little while, but first I want to discuss one way in which one's medical status goes out of control – waiting for test results. The scenario goes something like this:

- You get a diagnostic medical test.

- You then have to wait, often for unreasonable amounts of time, for the results.

- Each minute seems like an hour, and each hour seems like a lifetime. For you, time is suspended around one thing: the results.

- The lab staff and other medical personnel tell you that it takes time for the test results to come in, that the diagnostics need to be sent to a lab in a faraway land, and that the doctor has a busy schedule.

Many in the medical field believe that "patients waiting for results" is just a part of the office protocol and you just have to hunker down, bite the bullet, keep the faith and a stiff upper lip, and wait for the doctor to get back to you when it is convenient for him or her. So many patients comply with this nonsense, for a number of reasons, including feeling too intimidated by the medical system, wanting to be stoically brave, and thinking they have no options. I learned this the hard way when I had to wait a week before finding out my prognosis.

And that was sheer mental anguish.

Frankly, waiting a long amount of time is bogus. You have the right to know your test results quickly. Most results are in a lot sooner than medical staff would have you believe. With computers and databases, doctors can get results with the touch of a button. I have seen this with my own diagnostic test results. The truth is, you have much more power than you think in getting the results on your timeline, not the medical personnel's:

1. Determine how long of a wait is acceptable to you. Hint: a week is too long.

2. If you cannot wait, call the doctor's office and tell the staff that waiting a long time for test results is harmful to you psychologically and physically. Tell them you must know the results by a certain date.

3. If this method doesn't work, call the doctor's office repeatedly with the previously mentioned message.

In short, make a pest of yourself. The goal is to speak with your doctor or another doctor as soon as possible about the test results. Consider requesting the results by phone. This method isn't for everyone, but sometimes a phone call is better than waiting an entire week to see the doctor in person. You can still meet with your doctor in a week, but at least you will have your results.

Throughout the duration of the wait, do things that will relax you mentally and physically. For me it was sketching, watching movies.... oh, and Xanax. How each person handles the wait is different, so do whatever you can to cope.

Caveat: Throughout your self-advocacy, you do need to be as tactful as possible. However, you should be assertive, direct, and willing to overcome your fears to do what's right for you.

Remember, nobody can advocate in this arena better than you. All you need are courage, guts, perseverance, resilience, and passion for your cause. So whatever your situation, here are some tips to help make your loss of control seem more bearable and how you can feel that you've kept at least some of your control. Caregivers you trust need to know this information as well, as they are also your advocates.

Examination Room Anxiety

Waiting for the doctor to enter the examination room feels like a lifetime, and each minute feels like a year. By the time the doctor enters the room, the patient is so stressed out that he/she needs medical help just for wait-anxiety. I have been bold enough to tell nurses that the wait is too long. And, believe it or not, I've had satisfactory results. But there are other constructive ways to cope and to keep your stress level even-keeled. This involves creating a toolbox of activities and coping mechanisms to help you de-stress. Everyone has to find his or her own toolbox that will best suit his or her purposes.

De-stressing – Packing your Toolbox

These are what I do to de-stress and what I recommend as part of your toolbox while waiting in the waiting room and the examination room:

1. Bring a book or several magazines to read – Don't rely on the reading material at a doctor's office; bring what you want to read and make sure it will provide at least a few hours of reading.

2. Bring music – an MP3 player with headphones often do the trick against wait-anxiety.

3. Sketch or draw – It engrosses one's attention, and you need not be an artist to do this.

4. Deep breathing – Use the diaphragm to breathe in.

5. Meditate or repeat a certain mantra – Mine is "I'm powerful." Having a mantra helps alleviate the wait-anxiety and empowers you.

6. Choose words to help you cope with any aspect of the medical system – facing the medical world is difficult, especially if you had or are currently

suffering from an affliction. It helps to have at least 10 positive words that describe you or that you want to describe you, each on its own index card. After reading each word, reflect on what that word means to you. You can even write on the cards and hang them up anywhere that suits your purpose.

I also find this helps me prepare and cope with doctor's appointments. You can also bring them to doctor's appointments with you. My words are:

- Powerful
- Courageous
- Gutsy
- Resilient
- Perseverance
- Tough
- Steely
- Smart
- Savvy
- Empowered

Advocacy in the Hospital

ICU – INTENSIVE CARE UNIT. IT'S INTENSIVE, alright. But it's not a care unit. I should know: I am a patient here. Before my double mastectomy with reconstruction at a hospital with an excellent reputation, I am ecstatic to hear I will spend time in ICU. I believe ICU will give me specialized, individualized care. Instead, my experience is so horrific, that I could make a living selling t-shirts that say, "I was in ICU, and I lived to tell about it."

After visiting hours, during which I receive first-rate treatment, a night of hell begins. All night long, an inexperienced nurse keeps forgetting to check on me at the intervals the doctor had ordered. To make matters worse, the nurse keeps telling me every graphic detail about each ICU patient's condition. I'll spare you the gory details, but she finally whispers in my ear, "You're the *lucky* one. You are the only one getting out of here *alive*." At least she whispers. The ICU staff in an adjacent room is singing loudly, making fun of one of the patients who probably

won't make it. I cry, thinking of that person, lying there –
as I am lying there – strapped in – with a mocking song
being the last thing he or she hears.

By the time my family comes to see me during visiting
hours, the smoke and mirrors are back. By 8 a.m., the
"competent," "caring" staff have shown up for their day
shift, just in time to give visiting families and friends the
show of their lives. When my family brings up my
complaints about the previous night, the medical staff
assures them I have been delirious from all the medication
and I am exaggerating. Understandably, my doctors aren't
fooled. I tell them about what I heard and saw. Concerned,
they complain to the ICU staff about various
mistreatments. I am proud of myself: After advocating for
myself, I would receive better treatment that night.

Or so I think.

The second night is equally demoralizing. I wake up in the
middle of the night, parched with thirst, and in near-total
darkness. My bed is shoved into a dark corner, and I feel
as if I were in a closet. I am afraid. I call out for someone
to please get me water, but to no avail. I beg for water non-
stop for hours and plead for someone to help me because
I am now afraid that I will die of thirst. I keep begging for
help. No ICU staff shows up until visiting hours begin. The
ICU staff tells my family that the medications had once
again made me delirious. Had a friend or relative been

there that entire night to advocate for me, I could've taken a break from begging and allowed my companion to do the dirty work.

The day after the "I'm-Dying-From-Thirst-But-Nobody-Showed-Up-Last-Night" episode, I tell my surgeon what happened. He decides that although I am supposed to spend another night in ICU, it is detrimental for me to be there any longer, so I am moved to a far better unit, one without the words "Intensive Care" in it.

Night Sweats

Here's the truth: when the night staff starts their shift in the hospital, you can bet that you will receive poor care resulting from incompetent people. Oh, an occasional good doctor or medical assistant will pop by from time to time, but, rest un-assured, your evenings will yield no rest. Most likely you will be subject to a variety of staff members who won't know how to care for you or know how to care for you but are unwilling to, so in order to advocate for yourself, do the following:

- You must speak up.

- You must not be intimidated by the authority of medical personnel.

- If you cannot advocate for yourself, have someone available who can speak up on your behalf.

From my various stays in regular units, I've had to put up with a lot of neglect. Like the time I was in a post-lumpectomy surgical daze and had to tell medical personnel they were strapping the blood pressure cuff on the wrong arm. They admitted that they didn't know what surgery I had (look at the chart!) until I told them. All night, rather than resting, I argued with staff about their trying to put the blood pressure cuff on the wrong arm (look at the chart!). I finally had a big sign placed over my bed that identified the arm from which to take blood pressure (look at the sign!). The sign wasn't ever read, so instead of sleeping, I stayed on guard all night to keep reminding the staff of their jobs.

How about the time I was left to lie in my own body fluids leaking from drains, long after I called for a nurse to come in? Or the time medical staff pinned the front of my gown closed, but left the safety pins open so I was being stuck all night? When I complained, the staff couldn't find the source that was sticking me. I eventually found the open safety pins and fixed the problem.

There were also the numerous times staff didn't answer right away when I pressed my call button. A few times I tried to communicate that my IV was empty, and you'd think the alarm indicating this would have tipped them off. There were also instances when the medical staff forgot to hook up my pressure cuffs on my calves designed to prevent blood clots. I had to remind them to re-attach the cuffs and that this was vital to preventing blood clots. There was also a time when the measuring vessel I had to urinate in had someone else's urine in it. Did I mention that hospitals are filthy places, not conducive to healing? And I still remember the night when the nurses and medical assistants had a party right outside of my room. I told them I was trying to recover from surgery and that I'd appreciate it if they kept it down. They hated me. But they used their inside voices.

Advocating for yourself while you are in the hospital is especially difficult. You are already in a vulnerable state and sometimes in a post-surgery and/or under-medication daze. Whatever hospital unit you are in, I really cannot emphasize enough the importance of having an advocate — someone you know and trust — staying overnight with you or keeping a close eye on you, whatever unit you are in, but especially in ICU. Insisting you have someone there during the night won't win you popularity contests, but it will help ensure that you can avoid the trauma of the very unit that is supposed to take care of you.

Making the Most out of Your Hospital Stay Checklist

Here is the checklist that can help make your hospital stay more bearable:

✔ Don't allow your cell phone to be taken. After surgery, if the staff still doesn't allow cell phones, then make plans for someone to sneak it to you.

✔ Bring a cell phone with audio and video recording capabilities.

✔ R&R: Repeat and repeat often. Keep telling hospital staff your needs.

✔ Speak up or have your overnight advocate do so.

✔ Press call buttons until someone responds.

✔ Complain to doctors and day hospital staff if you felt you received subpar care during the night.

✔ Complain to anyone who will listen.

✔ Bring a care package, such as soothing music, a book, a sketchpad, etc. Don't be disappointed if you can't use any of them in your recovery process.

Out-patient Self-Advocacy

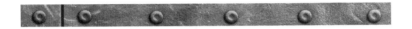

3.6% – THAT'S HOW MUCH MY BONE DENSITY
has increased over the past two years, launching me from
near-osteoporosis to near-normal bone density range. As
someone who has fought for my life, each victory counts.
The Dexa Scan, or bone-density scan, results are finally in
my favor. It has taken years of hard work to up the bone
density ante by 3.6%. Physicians tell me that my exercise
regimen, calcium supplements, and a medication designed
to increase bone-density have all helped.

I am joyful.

Rewind to a few years earlier.

A recent Dexa Scan shows a minor improvement in my
bone mass. I know the results are "good" from reading
the report, but being somewhat data challenged, I go to
a family practice doctor I am familiar with. My PCP isn't
in the office that day. Chemotherapy and its subsequent

premature menopause had left me struggling in the bone-density arena. At a young age, I found myself on the brink of osteoporosis. The doctor says of the improvement in my bone density, "These are significant numbers, but for a person as young as you, these are very, very bad results."

I am crushed.

All I want is a glimmer of hope. After all, bone density increasing is good news. And yet, he nearly reduces me to tears. Defiantly, I tell him I believe I can continue to increase my bone density further because I'm so proactive in my health. He stares at me blankly and says, "That's not going to happen. No matter what you do, your bones are going to continue to deteriorate. There's no place for you to go but down."

I leave the appointment depressed, without hope.

A few months later I ask my oncologist if it is possible to still gain bone density, and to my surprise he says, "Absolutely. It's very possible." I cling to that hope – the hope that I could play the hand I've been dealt as well as possible. And now, I have a 3.6% improvement in bone density. According to my gynecologist, "This is a significant gain. You are almost at the normal range."

Oh and about that doom-and-gloom doctor – he's so *fired*.

What I Learned:

It's very easy to get caught up in the idea that a doctor's word is as good as gold, when in reality, his or her viewpoint isn't necessarily the correct one. Feel free to fire such a doctor.

Patients need hope they can be healed, that they can have minimal suffering, that their families are there beside them, and so on. Many find solace in religious faith and/or in knowing that their loved ones are there to support them in time of a medical crisis. It is a doctor's responsibility to give you accurate information in a respectful manner and to offer solace without sugar coating anything. At the same time, a physician should not be overly pessimistic when it is not warranted.

There's no room for excess drama in a doctor's office. That should be saved for the plethora of medical dramas on TV.

Patient Self-Advocacy Checklist

To help advocate for yourself when you are sick, do the following:

✔ Collaborate in your medical care, viewing doctors as partners.

✔ Even if your life is spinning out of control, think of ways that your life is in control. Be mindful that, to some extent, you have control over your life.

✔ Assert your needs to your doctor.

✔ Use tools in your toolbox to help you cope in the waiting and examination rooms.

✔ If hospitalized, make sure your needs are being met.

✔ When in the hospital have a trustworthy person on hand to advocate for you, even if he or she can spend the night.

Fire any doctor who views your good medical news as something negative.

Part III – Closing Thoughts

It's important to regain a sense of control, even during the chaos of being a patient and especially during the chaos of being hospitalized. Hospital staff like nice, quiet, passive, non-complaining patients. But you will be the rabble rouser. You will make your voice heard. Your health, and possibly life, depends on it. You are too important to be immaterial to incompetent and uncaring hospital staff.

You matter.

Part IV:
CIVIL
DISOBEDIENCE

Civil Disobedience

Caveat:

DESPITE WHAT YOU'VE JUST READ, MANY OF THE medical staff I've encountered have been helpful and kind. Most of the time, my doctor visits have been made more pleasant and relaxing – all because of the administrative staff – such as receptionists, medical assistants, records people – who do have a difficult job and often have to deal with rude patients. However, this book is about how to deal with less-than-stellar medical staff and situations. So here it goes.

This book can help you stand up to rude medical personnel who seem bent on placing hurdles in your way or being rude and inappropriate during your visit to the office. I speak from experience, and I am grateful for these experiences because they taught me the incredible power patients have.

Doctors Behaving Badly – Part I

MY SURGEON BEAMS AS HE CHECKS OUT HIS handiwork, knowing that the mass he removed from my right breast was benign. He is joyful. He once again gets to save my breast. It doesn't seem to register to him that three surgeries to remove tissue have left my breast horribly deformed and still at risk for a breast cancer recurrence. I know that if I don't act now, something *will* go wrong. In fact, I feel that something is already wrong, but I can't identify it.

"I've decided to get a double mastectomy with reconstruction," I say. "I would like you to perform the double mastectomy."

"That won't be necessary," he says. "The mass was benign and I don't see the point in removing healthy breasts."

"But," I say, "Doctors say it's hard to tell what's going on in my breasts. I've already had breast cancer, and I know I will slip through the cracks if I don't remove both breasts."

"But your left breast is healthy. I don't believe in removing healthy breasts."

"But how do you know there aren't cancer cells in the left breast?"

"I can understand your fears, but there is no reason to remove healthy breasts. I don't agree with you. We'll monitor you closely instead."

Then a voice within me comes out. It is the voice of courage and self-preservation.

"No, I've made the decision already. They come off. Have you ever had a patient so in tune with her body and so keen with intuition, that she knew that if a procedure weren't done, that her life would be in jeopardy?"

"I don't have the intuition that you claim to have," he sneers. "Nor have I had patients whose intuition was correct. We can't work on intuition alone. There have to be facts, and the facts say that you have healthy breasts."

At this point I know he's not on board with me philosophically, and I have not achieved buy-in. I have to find another surgeon. While I feel empowered through my civil disobedience, I am also sad. The breast-conserving surgeon no longer serves my purposes. We must part ways. This heated conversation is the beginning of a yearlong fight for the double mastectomy. I ultimately get my way, and a biopsy shows that the left breast my former surgeon had deemed healthy is filled with precancerous cells.

What I Learned:

Even when facing a doctor armed with knowledge, I found that I was also armed with a valuable tool: the ability to speak up when my very life was at stake. Even though I was in dire medical straits with a real medical threat looming, I was able to fight for my rights as a medical patient – not only to have my voice be heard, but to bring about what I needed: the appropriate medical care, even if that meant being civilly disobedient.

The term "civil disobedience" is a long-used concept usually applied to encourage non-violent disobedience toward oppressive governments. I encourage you to apply this concept in the medical arena – civil disobedience against oppressive medical staff – from doctors to administrators. If it was good enough for Gandhi, it is good enough for you.

Let's face it: Those in the medical field have the upper hand in dealing with you because, well, being a patient is darn well intimidating and confusing. Navigating the medical system is daunting and difficult. For many, being a patient is a "career" of a sort because it either feels like or is a full-time job. In addition, those of you dealing with serious conditions probably feel as if your life is spinning out of control, as mentioned in Part III: *Advocacy When Sick.*

The last thing you need is abuse from medical staff.

To get your medical needs heard and met, you sometimes must practice civil disobedience against authority when appropriate. For example, if your gut instinct is telling you one thing, and a doctor is telling you another thing, speak up. If you don't see eye-to-eye with a physician or physician's assistant, speak up. Whether you are dealing with doctors, receptionists and/or records personnel don't hesitate to speak up.

Your life may depend upon it.

Doctors Behaving Badly – Part II

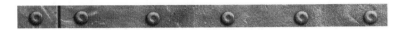

I SEE A SURGEON WHO SAYS MY DECISION FOR a preventive double mastectomy is medically sound and he is willing to perform the surgery, but a few weeks later, something goes awry. He tells me that breast cancer is associated with colon cancer, so before he does the surgery, I need a colonoscopy.

Huh?

He says that while the reconstructive surgeons are finishing the surgery, he also wants to remove my ovaries and uterus, as well. I initially like the idea of surgical double dipping or one-stop-shopping, if you will, for I think two fewer organs means two fewer organs to get cancer.

However, my PCP and oncologist both agree that I should not be under anesthesia for longer than the 10 hours the double mastectomy with reconstruction will take. They also say a colonoscopy is not necessary at this time. I defer to their expertise.

The surgeon is royally pissed off when he finds this out and keeps pushing to remove my ovaries and uterus. And his fixation with both organs is turning the focus of my surgery off its initial purpose – to hopefully prevent a breast cancer recurrence. He is more concerned with his ego than my health. I call the surgeon several times and leave messages for him to return my calls. I don't hear from him for a month. Then, one day, out of the blue, he calls me. He scolds me for not following *his* orders, making me feel horrible. He temporarily – and I mean temporarily – sets me back into hopelessness. I get yet *another* opinion with an oncology-gynecologist surgeon, whatever that is. The second-opinion guy also recommends removing the ovaries, but not the uterus or my getting a colonoscopy.

I am confused at this unfolding nightmare.

After a week of reflection, I realize having organ-removing enthusiasts on one's medical team is worse than having no doctor at all. Most importantly, I realize my organs are my own, my body is my own, and I have a strong say in my medical destiny; it is *my* decision which doctors to align myself with. I can hire and fire any doctor at will. I feel confident.

Ironically, the abusive surgeon wants to assist my team of doctors with the double mastectomy with reconstruction.

I insist, "No, I don't want his hands on me. In fact, I don't even want him near me during the surgery." My wishes are respected.

I feel powerful.

What I Learned:

In many cases, complying with a doctor's instructions makes sense. But when a physician insisted that I ignore my intuition, didn't take my concerns seriously, and bullied and mocked me, I needed to fight back and let my voice be heard. A doctor's competence is one thing. How he or she treats a patient is another matter altogether.

Some doctors try to silence you into blind compliance. These individuals do this through a variety of tactics, which include interrupting you, belittling you, minimizing your concerns, marginalizing you, and using their authority and expertise as the only truth.

These individuals shouldn't fare well with you.

When a doctor tries to destroy your autonomy and encourages you to ignore your intuition, you need to practice civil disobedience. Period. Many doctors like passive patients. Don't be that passive patient; instead, be assertive and speak up.

Cold Reception – Part I

I FEEL STRESS, ANGER, AND FRUSTRATION. I AM
waiting for pre-surgery bloodwork. My veins are ready
to cooperate – but the lab administrators are not. The
receptionist is rude, haughtily insisting I need a hard
copy referral – even though she has just printed out the
electronic version from my physician. The receptionist
then directs me to an even nastier intake person at
another desk, who coldly says the center can't do
labwork without a hard copy referral.

"But I'm having major surgery in a week, and my doctor
told me an electronic referral would suffice," I say. She
responds that the center would do the labwork, but only if
I sign a form agreeing to pay for the procedure should my
insurance not cover it – which is a possibility, according to
her, because the referral is electronic.

No, it doesn't make sense to me either.

She shoves the form toward me, and that's where my civil disobedience kicks in. I tell her, "You know, every time I come to this office, I am treated rudely and with disrespect. I *demand* respect. I followed the correct protocol. So I *refuse* to sign this form." I return the unsigned form to her.

Her eyes widen in shock that anyone would have the audacity to tell her this. She scribbles something on the form. I ask her what she is writing, and she says, "Patient refuses to sign form."

I get my blood-work that day and don't pay a cent.

When I tell my friends about my refusal to cooperate, they say they never knew they could refuse to sign a medical form. Well, now they – and you – know. While we should treat medical staff with respect, when we find ourselves bullied by them, we should not passively comply. We should be civilly disobedient.

A few years later, I experience déjà vu at a different lab. This time, the patient is my daughter, who needs routine lab work. The lab had previously informed me that all I needed to do was provide the doctor's order for the test to be conducted and that I did not need a referral.

When I bring the order in, the registration receptionist tells me I need a referral from the doctor – not merely an order. And she is on some super nasty power trip. She then hands me a form that looks all-too-familiar; it is the same form I refused to sign when getting my pre-surgery blood work, the form that says because there is no referral, I agree to pay whatever insurance doesn't cover.

"I refuse to sign this," I say. "You can easily get a referral, so there's no way I'd ever pay for lab work that is covered by my insurance."

She says, "What? This form just says you acknowledge you don't have a referral."

"But that's *not* what this form says," I reply. "This form says that I will have to pay any costs if there is no referral. And I refuse to pay. In fact, rather than signing the form, I'm going to write on it an explanation of why this office has led me astray."

Now *she's* in shock, as I write about the situation and how the lab registration personnel led me astray and never told me about a referral in the first place. I also write that my not having a referral is the fault of the lab staff who have also caused me a major inconvenience. For good measure, I add, "I will not pay for services rendered because I had a doctor's order for the lab tests and followed the proper protocol." I then sign that what I just wrote is true.

Cold Reception – Part II

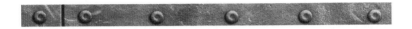

I'M IN MY SURGEON'S WAITING ROOM WITH strangers, wondering whether I will have a future. An MRI has shown a possible breast cancer recurrence, and I am doing everything possible not to cry. It has been a rough year: My dear friend died young of breast cancer, and I am now wondering whether I will share the same fate.

Suddenly, the receptionist calls me up to the front desk and loudly says that I owe a certain amount of money and asks whether I want to pay it now. I am in such a state of panic regarding my health that I don't even remember whether I even owe money or how much. Considering all I have been through lately, cutting a check isn't at the forefront of my concerns. Barely audible, I meekly tell her I need to see the bill and that I will pay it eventually. She then tells me to sit down. I return to my seat, feeling depressed, defeated, and publicly humiliated.

And then I get angry.

I go back up to the receptionist and say, "You know, I might have a possible breast cancer recurrence, and I can't believe you want to discuss my bill at a time like this!" Before she can stop stammering, I add, "You and anyone in your office are *never, ever* to discuss anything bill-related with me in this office." She manages an apology.

I return to my seat, still feeling sad, but now empowered.

After visiting with the surgeon and in the process of making an appointment for a biopsy, I break down and sob bitterly, tears falling from my sleep-deprived eyes. The nurse comforts me. Had the incident with the receptionist not occurred, I might have broken down anyway, but let's face it: her inappropriate timing and insensitivity hasn't helped matters.

What I Learned:

Facing receptionists can sometimes be as intimidating as facing physicians. Despite my fears, when treated harshly by medical administrative staff, I found the ability to speak up on my behalf. When facing administrative personnel, the same rules apply as when facing abusive doctors: speak up, don't give up.

Sometimes advocacy takes a simple path. Simple enough that all it requires is to tell a doctor's nasty receptionist to basically shut up. We have HIPAA rights and sign a zillion forms attesting to these rights. But what about the receptionist who announces your business – from medical to financial – loud enough for everyone in the waiting room to hear it? Financially speaking, it's only right to pay what you owe, even if it's in installments. What's wrong is if receptionists handle it publicly.

No matter your medical circumstances, you can summon up enough courage to stick up for yourself when confronted by an intimidating receptionist. *Never* give up and don't allow fear and intimidation to rule you. When a staff member in a doctor's office announces your business in a public place, it is *your* business to speak up and tell that person how rude he/she is being and/or inform the doctor of this problem. When dealing with a potential or existing medical problem, the last thing you need to hear is a medical staff member discussing extraneous/money matters with you. This type of insensitivity to your needs is unacceptable.

Remember, *you* call the shots in how you are treated – and as the patient you deserve to be treated with respect.

You are your own best advocate. Don't tolerate rudeness from medical and administrative personnel. You have the right to be respected as a human being. That means not being rushed through an appointment, talked down to, not being manipulated and made to feel guilty, sorry, inferior, disillusioned, marginalized, minimalized, and the list goes on and on.

In an ideal world, medical personnel are allies in your care. Unfortunately, all too often, medical staffs are opponents and annoying hindrances. Some doctors and nurses are rude, not counting the administrators, the "gatekeepers" of a frustrating bureaucratic system. While you should be civil to any medical opponent (aka not swearing or threatening them to a dueling match), you can use your actions and words to sting like a bee, wasp, or any other insect of your choice.

Make Sure the Doctor You See is the One You're Supposed to See

I have a stress fracture on my right foot. My primary care physician refers me to an orthopedic surgeon who, incidentally, no longer works on breaks in the feet. So I call her to get a referral to another orthopedic surgeon. She isn't in the office, but another doctor says he will handle the referral. I call the office of the referred specialist and was all set to make the appointment, when suddenly, THE question popped into my head: I asked the receptionist, "This doctor is an orthopedic surgeon, right?" And she stumbled over her words and said, "No, he's a foot doctor." I asked her to clarify what this meant, and it turns out he is a podiatrist, NOT an orthopedic surgeon.

I have nothing against podiatrists, but in the case of my stress fracture, my primary care physician wants me to see an orthopedic surgeon. I call her office back and complain.

The receptionist says that if this other doctor referred me to a podiatrist, there must have been a good reason for it. And I say, "Well, he's in no position to determine what kind of specialist is best for me. My PCP wanted me to see an orthopedic surgeon for a reason." The receptionist sounds shocked. My PCP calls me back as soon as she can, and she finds the right orthopedic surgeon for me.

What I Learned

The whole medical run-around is even more cracked than a stress fracture, and I found as a patient I had to take a stand when appropriate. We all deserve the best medical care possible. That's why it's important to ask the follow-up question of a lifetime: the one verifying that the doctor you are setting an appointment to see is, indeed, the one whom you are supposed to see.

While many in administration are nice and comply with your needs, many others are not, and these are the ones I'm focusing on. And while many doctor's assistants and nurse practitioners are highly competent, the bottom line is this: You have *the right* to see the doctor, not an assistant, if that is your will. And that means assertiveness and focus. After all, what is your insurance or your own pocket paying for?

You must be persistent by plowing through all the nonsense that unfeeling or uncaring medical staff throws at you. In the aforementioned situation/scenario, it would've been easier for me to be complacent, but in the long run it would not have been the right choice. Often the things we know are worth having – like appointments with quality doctors you know (or want to get to know) and trust – are worth fighting for. You have to sometimes repeat yourself and your key ideas/phrases to get what you want and need.

This is the routine we hate, don't we? Dealing with receptionists and other administrators who seem born to make your life difficult. These people, perhaps overworked or given orders from somewhere to cut corners, try to give you an appointment with a nurse's assistant or a physician's assistant when it's clear you want and need to see the doctor.

When it comes to advocating for yourself, you must sometimes be willing to shamelessly share your situation in the public arena. This is because medical staff and each of us have limited availability, and, well, you sometimes have to snatch that narrow window of time you have to make that call.

This is exactly what happened to me.

Just for the Records – Part I

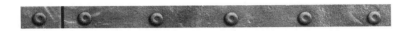

THE DRAMA UNFOLDS WITH ME AS LEAD ACTOR, director, and writer of my medical destiny – oh, and a train car packed with complete strangers who have no idea that their ticket purchases to downtown Chicago include entertainment. Well, that day, they get a lot of bang for their buck.

I have an appointment with a mastectomy surgeon the next day. Her office has squeezed me in quickly, as my surgery date is in a month. I just find out about the appointment that very morning. Understandably, this surgeon's office needs my medical records faxed from another doctor's office ASAP. It takes a 45-minute phone fight, with me as victor, and, as it turns out, a crowd of strangers cheering for me.

Here's how my drama unfolded that very eventful day

Needing my records faxed and knowing I'd be unavailable the entire afternoon, I make the call while on the train. The records person is refusing to fax my records to the surgeon's office. By the time I make the call, I am pissed off, tired, and my frustration has turned to steely determination. The records administrator says it normally takes a week or two to transfer medical records, and then she scolds me. She says I am asking the impossible: the office to fax records the day before the appointment. She adds that I should know better. I calmly explain that the mastectomy surgeon's office fit me in at the last minute because of the urgency of my medical situation and *that's* why I need the records delivered on such short notice. I just found out this morning, I explain, that I am seeing her tomorrow.

To my dismay, the records lady counters that there are protocols to follow and that the office can't just fax records willy-nilly whenever a patient asks for them. I remind her that the surgeon is the one who wants to see me immediately and wants my medical records before my appointment. The administrator says her office's policy is strict, and if they make an exception for me, then they are going to have to make it for every patient. So sorry, but no tumbling dice.

I say, "OK" and end the conversation. I cry quietly – after all, it's OK for the whole train car to know my breasts are coming off, but I don't want anyone seeing me cry. (I am train car-decorum-challenged.) I feel defeated. But I call the office again. The record keeper recognizes my voice and is amazed I have the audacity to come back for more abuse. As she starts telling me her office's decision is final, I interrupt her with a *blitzkrieg* of my own: "I don't want to speak with *you* anymore. Give me your office manager."

Shocked at my irreverence, she complies.

When the office manager gets on the phone, she tells me she cannot go against office protocol regarding sending records to a doctor's office. Suddenly, I take a different approach: emotional manipulation, and this is the turning point that gives me the upper hand in getting what I want and need.

Seeming to change the subject, I say, "Do you know I'm adopting a baby girl from China?"

"Awww, how sweet!"

"Well, how would you feel if she no longer had her mommy?"

"That would be terrible!"

"Well, that will happen if I don't get my surgery. Your office's refusal to deliver my medical records today may delay my surgery and ultimately harm me. How would you like to tell my daughter that she no longer has a mommy?"

"Please don't talk that way! We don't want your child to be motherless. Let me see what I can do to get your records to the surgeon's office."

I thank her and two minutes later — no I really mean literally two minutes — the person I initially had spoken with humbly calls me back and says the records have just been faxed to the surgeon's office. My surgeon's office calls me a few minutes later to confirm this.

I am exiting the train in shock at my own power to advocate for myself — and in shock that I'm able to stand on trembling legs. And as I walk on shaky legs, but not on shaky ground anymore, I think that perhaps I became someone's role model and hero that day. And I realize I have become my own hero that day, as well.

Just for the Records – Part II

THE MAMMOGRAPHY TECHNICIANS ARE KIND AND easy to work with. Unfortunately they have nothing to do with ensuring my records are ready on time. I'm always supposed to pick up my mammogram films and report right before I see my surgeon. He wants to see them during my routine visits, so I always call the records department ahead of time to tell the personnel that I am coming to pick them up. Yes, even though the hospital has a courier service, I have to physically go and pick them up and then head to my appointment the day of the appointment.

Now this is the shocker: about 50% of the time the mammography results aren't ready, and I have to go to the doctor without the mammogram film and report, which usually arrives at the surgeon's office a few days later. With dense breast tissue, I am afraid I am going to slip through the cracks. Besides, I hate waiting for the surgeon to call me post-appointment to tell me the mammogram results, rather than getting the results the day of the appointment. For someone who has been through cancer, or any harrowing medical experience for that matter, waiting a few days is like waiting an eternity. And to further complicate matters at this mammography center, whichever individual happens to be at the front desk is always rude and cold to me. I find this intimidating and the first few times I use this outpatient service, I passively tolerate their mistreatment and utter disrespect.

After being a relatively passive patient the first two years after treatment, I finally call the outpatient mammography and lab center to complain about the mishandling of these mammograms and, after speaking to several impolite personnel, I finally get a friendly staff member. I tell her that since I already had breast cancer and have dense breast tissue, my mammograms need careful inspection by my surgeon **on time** and that such mishaps could one day cost me my life.

She says flippantly, "Aw, honey, you're not likely to get breast cancer again."

I volley back: "How do *you* know that? You can't tell a patient *that*! It is vital that your office ensures prompt and accurate delivery of my mammogram films and results."

After about two years of nearly slipping through the cracks with the mammography results, I finally assert myself to my surgeon – I politely insist that, with my history of breast cancer, it isn't prudent for me to get follow-up mammograms at an unreliable place. The stakes are too high, I explain, to allow this kind of incompetence to determine my medical fate. From this point on, I want my mammograms done at the hospital's far superior breast center. I get buy-in from him: He agrees, regularly writes referrals to the specialty breast center, and I never have such problems again.

What I Learned:

Like most patients, getting records departments to cooperate on my behalf seemed insurmountable. The stakes are always too high to allow the incompetence of mediocre record keepers to interfere with my medical outcomes. Nobody should have to endure this sloppy treatment from records departments.

Records departments simply amaze me. They are able to provide services and obtain records lickety-split when a doctor requests them, but not when a patient does. Getting records transferred from one physician's office to another is really easy, but all the red tape can seem insurmountable to a patient. For those with managed-care plans, the step from getting a referral to seeing a specialist is fraught with hurdles.

We all want to have our discussions with medical personnel to be confidential and private. But sometimes we don't have that luxury, especially with the lack of sensitivity medical personnel sometimes have toward our time constraints. They call you back on *their* time. You should seize the reins in how records get delivered, and you need to be proactive in following through. If you don't, nobody else will. Don't wait for the records to get to the doctor's office. Call your doctor's office to determine whether it received records. If not, pick them up in person.

With steely perseverance and determination, you can get what *you* want, no matter how difficult or impossible it seems. When confronted with rude medical staff bent on making your visit miserable, there's only one good option: Civil Disobedience.

Civil Disobedience Checklist

To practice civil disobedience, be mindful of the following:

✔ Don't allow doctors and administrative staff to intimidate you into blind compliance.

✔ Make sure you keep an eye on medical records departments, for they won't keep an eye on you.

Part IV – Closing Thoughts

Doctors and medical administration can behave badly and it is up to you, the patient, to keep them in line. In particular, records departments can be very uncooperative. The key is to be persistent and proactive to get the care and follow-through you so need and deserve. At the beginning of the book, I provided my version of what a patient-centered bill of rights should look like. Here it is again.

PATIENT'S BILL OF RIGHTS

1. You have the right to be civilly disobedient with any medical personnel who you perceive does not have your best interest at heart.

2. You have the right to hire and fire doctors at will.

3. You have the right to question treatments without a doctor being condescending to you.

4. You have the right to understand you are on equal footing with a doctor because you are both human beings with comparable self-worth.

5. You have the right to collaborate with excellent doctors you trust and who truly have your best interest at heart.

6. You have the right to a voice in your own medical care.

7. You have a right to have doctors return your phone calls on a timely basis.

8. You have the right to follow your gut instinct and not allow medical people to manipulate you into ignoring it.

9. Whether you are incapacitated, in the hospital, or extremely sick, you have the right to speak up in any medical settings.

10. You have the right to choose your medical destiny to whatever extent possible.

11. You have the right not to be bullied or badgered by anyone – from receptionist to doctor – at any time.

12. You have the right to be treated with respect and to employ civil disobedience if you are being bullied, badgered, and disrespected in any way. In short, say "no" to thugs.

This book isn't about ignoring doctors' orders, which often are sound. However, letting your guard down in the medical arena can be a costly mistake. You have the right to be properly informed about your medical situation and to be treated with respect. Doctors, nurses, and other medical personnel are not perfect, and, being human like everyone else, they can and do make mistakes. Unfortunately, some are unaware what is in your best interest, and that's why it's more important than ever to take charge of your medical care, which includes seeking out whatever resources possible. Ultimately, *you* call the shots in your medical care.

Many of us learn to trust and obey all authority figures, including doctors. In fact, many of us view doctors as heroes. Many doctors are, indeed, heroes, but they are also human beings who can err. We forget that. This is part of why we sometimes ignore our own self-preservation instincts. Almost all members of the animal kingdom act on pure instinct to protect themselves and their loved ones. All except one: Humans. Far too often, humans deliberately trade their survival instincts for vulnerability – all because of an intimidating medical system. Your goal is to get what you need and deserve: great medical care and respect from medical personnel. You need to hone in on what you need and deserve and then go for it with all your energy.

My breast cancer experience transformed me from a meek, passive patient to an assertive one. As I have become bolder with the medical system, I still find self-advocacy really unpleasant. I usually am afraid whenever I walk into a doctor's office. But I am courageous, which means I act on my behalf in spite of my fears. And I tend to garner respect from medical personnel. It's a myth that only fearless, brash people can effectively advocate for themselves. It's a myth that you have to be outgoing to tell medical staff what's what. It's a myth that having courage means being fearless.

You can advocate for yourself. All you have to do is tap deep within you and act. And you will be the ordinary person who does the extraordinary. You are powerful enough to effectively advocate for yourself and loved ones.

And know your hero. It is not your doctor. It is *you*.

Made in the USA
Charleston, SC
07 July 2016